MUSCLE BUILDING

Proven Step by Step Guide to Get the Body You Always Dream About

John Carter

© **Copyright 2016 by John Carter- All rights reserved.**

This document is geared towards providing exact and reliable information in regards to the topic and issue covered. The publication is sold with the idea that the publisher is not required to render accounting, officially permitted, or otherwise, qualified services. If advice is necessary, legal or professional, a practiced individual in the profession should be ordered.

- From a Declaration of Principles which was accepted and approved equally by a Committee of the American Bar Association and a Committee of Publishers and Associations.

In no way is it legal to reproduce, duplicate, or transmit any part of this document in either electronic means or in printed format. Recording of this publication is strictly prohibited and any storage of this document is not allowed unless with written permission from the publisher. All rights reserved.

The information provided herein is stated to be truthful and consistent, in that any liability, in terms of inattention or otherwise, by any usage or abuse of any policies, processes, or directions contained within is the solitary and utter responsibility of the recipient reader. Under no circumstances will any legal responsibility or blame be held against the publisher for any reparation, damages, or monetary loss due to the information herein, either directly or indirectly.

Respective authors own all copyrights not held by the publisher.

The information herein is offered for informational purposes solely, and is universal as so. The presentation of the information is without contract or any type of guarantee assurance.

The trademarks that are used are without any consent, and the publication of the trademark is without permission or backing by the trademark owner. All trademarks and brands within this book are for clarifying purposes only and are the owned by the owners themselves, not affiliated with this document.

Table of Contents

Introduction 5

Chapter 1: The Need for More Muscles 6

Chapter 2: The Science of Building Muscle 9

Chapter 3: Exercising for Muscle Growth Part I 11

Chapter 4: Exercising for Muscle Growth Part II 18

Chapter 5: Exercising for Muscle Growth Part III 25

Chapter 6: Weight Lifting Tips for Maximum Muscles 34

Chapter 7: Eating for Muscle Growth 53

Conclusion 57

Introduction

I want to thank you and congratulate you for purchasing the book, *Muscle Building – Proven Step by Step Guide to Get the Body You Always Dream About.*

This book contains proven steps and strategies on how you can successfully build more muscle, which is very important in many different areas of life. Here, I'll discuss the 3 main ingredients for muscle building – training, rest and recuperation, and nutrition. And the best part is that I wont' overwhelm you – this book provides enough information to build muscle mass without overwhelming you. You will actually be encouraged to start! And by the end of this book, you'll be on your way to start building serious muscle mass!

Thanks again for purchasing this book, I hope you enjoy it!

Chapter 1: The Need for More Muscles

So why do you need to build more muscle mass? I can think of at least 9 reasons to do so. The first reason is having more muscle increases your metabolism. Why? It's because skeletal muscle, which is considered to be metabolically active. Simply put, the more muscle mass you build, the more calories should be able to burn on a daily basis. And when you workout your muscles hard, you also enjoy the benefit of burning significantly more calories during the recovery phase, i.e., while resting! Really, it's not that complicated. All you need to do is exert enough effort in your strength training.

Second, strengthening your muscles can help make your bones, tendons, and ligaments stronger. When this happens, you can significantly reduce your risks for injuries that can happen due to sports competition, playing around with your kids, training, or even just doing ordinary everyday things.

Third, gaining more skeletal muscle makes you look more fit, toned, and sexy. You can eventually lose body fat and look good, which can make you feel more confident about yourself, confident wearing great swim wear at the beach or the pool, and you'll be confident enough to wear practically any piece of clothing that you'd like to. Simply put, muscle is more aesthetically pleasing than fat.

Fourth, building more muscle mass also helps you perform cardiovascular workouts much better. It is your muscles that move your body and when you do cardio, you workout your muscles harder than you usually do. When that happens, you're working out your cardiovascular system.

Lifting weights even for just 20 minutes can be a much better cardiovascular workout then brisk walking for about an hour around the neighborhood. Plus lifting weights burns significantly more calories not just during the workout session itself but also even after exercise session.

Fifth, the more muscle mass you have, the higher your chances of living much longer. Tufts University discovered that the chances of living longer are much higher the more muscle mass a person has. It appears that muscle mass, and not cholesterol or blood pressure, was the barometer for longevity.

Sixth, more muscle mass can significantly increase the number of your body's insulin receptor sites. What this means is that you can make it easier for your body to stay lean and keep body fat levels to a minimum.

Seventh, building more muscle mass can help you improve your posture. This is because you need good body strength to hold good posture and to have good body strength you obviously need more muscle mass. Another benefit, which is attached to good body posture? Reduced risk or incidences of chronic pain from back problems such as sciatica.

Eighth, having more muscles makes performing daily activities much easier. When you have more muscle mass you become stronger, making it easier for you to lift things and perform certain movements. And with more muscle mass and strength, the better you're able to combat fatigue because it also helps increase your stamina.

Lastly, strength training helps you fight sarcopenia, which is a loss of muscle tissue due to aging. Unfortunately, the older we become, the less muscle mass we have. Between the ages of 20 to 90 years old, we may lose as much as 50% of our muscle mass. Women who are in menopause between the ages of 40 to 50 years old are estimated to lose about 1% muscle mass annually. And worse, lost muscle is usually replaced with body fat. Not exactly a favorable trade.

Carrying too much body fat can bring along with it many health issues. But when it comes to carrying more muscle mass, I haven't heard of any negative effects. So what does this mean? Building more muscle isn't something that you need to be afraid of. Therefore, you should strive to prioritize an exercise or training program that builds or at least maintains current muscle mass levels.

Chapter 2: The Science of Building Muscle

Before you can build muscles, you'll first need to understand the science behind it. And the more you understand the science, the better you'll be able to optimize muscle growth.

To build muscles, you must learn how to tear down and build up. What does this mean?

Have you ever suffered from a fractured bone? If you haven't, don't worry. You don't need to suffer from 1 to build muscle. My only point in asking if you suffered from a fracture before is that building muscle is similar to the recovery process involved in fractures.

When a bone is fractured or broken, it becomes much stronger than it was before, once fully healed. It's the same for muscles. Muscle growth happens when you tear down muscle fibers during exercise and in the healing or recovery process, they produce more muscle fibers that lead to more muscle mass. Again, such tears in muscle fibers aren't severe enough to injure you, as they are very small or only micro tears.

To you a clearer picture, let's imagine that your right bicep muscle is composed of 20,000 muscle fibers. Let's imagine that when you exercise your right bicep with the right kind of exercise, you will tear down about 500 muscle fibers. If you rest and eat properly after training, your right bicep muscle will compensate and recover by reproducing more muscle fibers than 500 that you tore down via exercise. In this imaginary example, you have an idea of how muscle building occurs with the right exercise and the right nutrition.

In order for you to successfully build muscle, you will need to consider the Holy Trinity of exercise, nutrition, and rest. If you get all of these three components right, you'll provide your muscles the optimal environment to grow.

So let's begin with exercise.

Chapter 3: Exercising for Muscle Growth Part I

Generally speaking, exercises may be classified into 3 different types, depending on the effect on the body: aerobic, anaerobic and flexibility. Aerobic exercises include walking, running, biking, hiking and any other exercises that are performed continuously for at least 20 minutes, the goal of which is to build up cardiovascular endurance. Anaerobic exercises include weight training, isometric exercises, and plyometric exercises that help improve muscular strength and increase muscle mass. Flexibility exercises, as the name suggests, help improve the body's flexibility, i.e., increase the muscles and joints' range of motion.

AEROBIC EXERCISES

Also referred to as cardio, the shorthand term for cardiovascular because of the cardiovascular benefits attributed to such, aerobic exercises are those that help make your body more efficient in terms of consuming oxygen. The word "aerobic" literally means "with oxygen", which is the consumption of oxygen as part of the body's energy generation or metabolic process.

There are many kinds of aerobic exercises, such as those I mentioned earlier. But the common thread they all have is that they are performed at moderate intensity levels for at least 20 minutes straight, which is at about 50%-80% of optimal heart rate.

The key here is continuous. If you play singles tennis and move continuously all throughout the game that is aerobic. But if you play doubles, where you have more frequent periods of non-activity compared to bursts of action, then it isn't aerobic anymore.

Aerobic exercises benefit your body in many ways. First, it makes your heart stronger. Being stronger helps make your heart become even more efficient in pumping blood all throughout your body – and oxygen is carried in the blood! So the more blood is circulated, the more oxygen your body's cells get – including your muscles! A stronger heart also brings down your resting heart rate.

Another benefit is better breathing. Aerobic exercises train your lungs so that they become stronger, which helps your body get more oxygen and breathe out carbon dioxide much faster.

Aerobic exercises also make your muscles healthier. Mind you, I said healthier, not bigger. How? Aerobic exercises help promote the growth of capillaries – or tiny blood vessels – in your muscles. With more blood vessels, there's more blood flowing in your muscles. And remember how oxygen is carried? That's right, by the blood! With more blood in the muscles, there's more oxygen, lower blood pressure, and minimize or remove metabolic wastes from the muscles, such as lactic acid.

Aerobic exercises help build stamina. While aerobics will make you somewhat tired while doing it and immediately after, your general stamina will eventually increase and you'll find yourself taking more and more time before you get tired doing physical activities.

Another benefit of aerobic exercise is in terms of weight. Performed correctly and with proper nutrition, aerobic exercises can also assist in healthy weight loss.

Aerobic exercises don't just make you fitter, they also help make you much healthier and live longer. For one, it helps you maintain a healthy weight, which significantly lowers your risks for ailments such as cancer, diabetes, stroke, high blood pressure and heart diseases. Performing weight-bearing aerobics like walking or running can also help you reduce your risks for osteoporosis, including its complications. And if you have arthritis, low or no-impact aerobics like swimming or biking help you maintain excellent cardiovascular fitness and a healthy body weight without straining or jarring your joints.

Another way aerobics help make you healthier is it's perceived ability to strengthen the immune system. It's believed that those who perform regular exercises, including aerobic ones, are less vulnerable to viral sicknesses like flu, colds and cough. A possible explanation for this is that aerobic exercises tend to assist the body in activating the immune system, which is what fights off infections.

Lastly, aerobic exercises don't just help you be physically healthy and fit – they also help you stay mentally healthy and fit! Doing such exercises help the body release the body's natural painkillers – endorphins. This hormone also helps bring down stress and to some extent, reduce depression and anxiety.

ANAEROBIC EXERCISE

This kind of exercise is one that helps you become stronger (more power) and build muscles. Training muscles anaerobically helps improve short-duration, high intensity activities that can last up to 2 minutes.

The most popular form of anaerobic exercise is strength training, which uses resistance to muscular contractions or movements, which results in the micro tears in muscles that I explained in Chapter 2 earlier. Ultimately, this results in stronger and bigger muscles.

Strength training comes in different forms, the most popular of which use weights and resistance. Weight and resistance exercises both utilize gravity (via dumbbells, barbells, kettle bells, etc.) or machines designed specifically to create resistance to muscular contraction such as bull bars, resistance bands, and the like.

When performed well, strength training exercises can give meaningful functional, overall health, and well being benefits. These include stronger ligaments, tendons, bones and muscles, improved endurance, tougher body, better joint movement, lower injury risks related to weak muscles, elevated levels of healthy cholesterol, and better cardiac functioning. Even better, such training helps maintain or increase lean body mass, which is key to healthy weight levels as well as reduced risk for developing osteoporosis later in life.

AEROBIC OR ANAEROBIC?

Regular aerobic exercise has been clearly shown to minimize the risk for or even treat serious chronic medical conditions that are life threatening such as depression, insomnia, Type-2 diabetes, heart diseases, obesity and high blood pressure. On the other hand, anaerobic exercises provide the body with continuous calorie-burning (metabolic) benefits that can continue long after the exercise session has been finished – up to 24 hours post exercise! Anaerobic exercises don't provide much of the benefits of aerobic ones and vice versa. But both help make the heart more efficient in different ways: aerobic exercises help increase cardiac volume and anaerobic exercises increase myocardial thickness.

So which is which: aerobic or anaerobic?

If the goal is general fitness is the goal, aerobic exercises simply won't cut it. General fitness requires a balanced training program and particularly, one that involves the development of muscular strength and endurance. But anaerobic exercise alone won't cut it either because the pathways that are used during metabolism in such exercises – particularly lactic acid fermentation and glycosis – that create the needed energy for low duration but high intensity exercises aren't utilized optimally. That's why aerobic exercises are also needed if the goal is simply general fitness.

If your goal is weight loss, specifically fat loss, it's worth noting that contrary to popular opinion, aerobics isn't the optimal exercise. Why? It's because it doesn't increase the body's basal metabolic rate (resting metabolism) as much as specific forms of anaerobic exercises. It can, however, be a good supplement to anaerobic training that gives that extra fat-burning kick.

Given that anaerobic exercises – particularly resistance exercises – are the ones that facilitate muscles growth, it should be your primary form of exercise for building muscle. You can learn a great deal from body builders like Arnold

Schwarzenegger, Flex Lewis, and the current best bodybuilder on earth, Phil Heath. All of them only perform aerobic exercises weeks before major contests like the Mr. Olympia in order to shed body fat and get really ripped.

Chapter 4: Exercising for Muscle Growth Part II

Now that you know you should make anaerobic or weight lifting/resistance training should be the foundation of your exercise program for building muscle, it's time to look into it further. In particular, let's take a look at 2 primary types of weight lifting or resistance movements: Compound and isolation exercises.

ISOLATION EXERCISES

Also referred to as single-joint exercises, these are exercises that move a single joint or muscle through a particular range of motion. How do isolation exercises look like? One is the bicep curl, which only involves moving, well, the bicep muscle on a single joint – the elbow. Another good example of an isolation exercise is leg extensions. As you straighten your legs, you only use the quadriceps or "quads" – as they're popularly called by weight lifting enthusiasts – and involve only the knee joint.

Lastly, one of the most popular isolation exercises are the side laterals, where you bring dumbbells from your hips upward to the sides up to shoulder level. This exercise involves only the shoulder joint and the only muscle that moves is the side deltoid or shoulder muscle.

COMPOUND EXERCISES

Also referred to as multi-joint exercises, they're clearly the opposite of isolation exercises in that these involve moving multiple muscles and joints through multiple ranges of motion. An example of this is the classic muscle building exercise – the bench press. Regardless if you're using a barbell or a pair of dumbbells, pressing the weight upward involves several muscles – primarily the chest muscles and secondarily the triceps muscles. It also works out your abs, lower back and rib muscles to stabilize both your body and the weight you're lifting. It also involves several joints - the shoulder joints and the elbow joints.

Another great example of a compound exercise is the squat. Regardless if you're using a barbell, a pair of dumbbells or a Smith machine, you work out several muscles and involve multiple joints. For the muscles, you contract the quadriceps, the calf and even the hamstrings. The joints involved in executing a squat include the hip, the knee, and the ankle joints. The squat also works out the biggest muscle group – the legs – and therefore burns the most calories!

Another great example of a compound exercise is the military or overhead press. As you press the weight upward and above your head, you work out the front deltoid (shoulder) muscles, your trapezius muscles (traps), and triceps muscles. You also move the shoulder and elbow joints to execute the overhead pressing movement.

MUSCLE GROWTH: ISOLATION OR COMPOUND?

Muscles grow – as I wrote in Chapter 2 – through the holy trinity of exercise, nutrition and rest. And if you examine the exercise part further, you'll remember that it's anaerobic or weight lifting/resistance training that allows your muscle fibers to tear and eventually rebuild and multiply, which leads to muscle growth.

Mechanical or muscular tension is key to creating the necessary micro tears in your muscle fibers so that it will reproduce even more fibers to grow. Simply put the more tension you apply to your muscles, the stronger and bigger they become. To this extent, you'll need to integrate or use as many muscles as you can if you hope apply the most tension on your muscles. That's why for muscle growth, the best lifting exercises are compound exercises.

Consider the chest muscle and two exercises: the barbell bench press (compound) and chest dumbbell flies (isolation). When it comes to the amount of weight you can use for the dumbbell flies, it's at most just half the weight you can hoist when you do barbell presses. Why? It's because with barbell presses, you involve more muscles and more joints. You don't put all the stress on just one joint and muscle. And given the principle that muscles will only grow when you exercise with great tension applied or heavy weights lifted, it makes sense that compound exercises are key to rapidly building muscle mass.

STRENGTH: ISOLATION OR COMPOUND?

What is strength? It's the ability to lift heavy weight. Hence, the stronger you are, the more weight you can lift. And to be able to lift really heavy weights, you need to integrate as many muscles and joints as you possibly can. This means you need to train primarily with compound exercises. Lifting the heaviest weight you can with isolation exercises simply won't allow you to develop as much strength as compound ones because it doesn't challenge your central nervous system as much. I don't want to drown you in too much technicality but believe me, the central nervous system needs to be challenged enough to force your muscles to adapt and become strong and when you perform compound exercises with heavy weight, you're able to do that.

ATHLETICISM: ISOLATION OR COMPOUND?

If no man is an island, the same holds true for your body parts – they don't exist separate from other parts. Every part of your body – bones, tendons, joints and muscles – are all part of a grander design that is your body. People only started to "isolate" body parts by defining each and every one of them as singular parts is for purposes of studying how the whole body works.

That being said, the body is always considered as one large system for movement rather than separate and smaller ones. When you look at it from that perspective, you begin to see that joints and muscles don't operate separately. Our bodies were designed to be a complex system of joints and muscles from top to bottom. True movement is therefore dependent on multiple joints and muscles working together.

Athleticism is your ability to perform movements that are, well, athletic! These include the ability to run, jump and move fast. And such movements require many different muscles and joints to execute. Have you ever tried jumping using your calf muscles only? Have you ever tried shooting a basketball from the 3-point line with just a flick of the wrist and nothing more? Or how about avoiding a football or rugby tackle with just your thigh muscle? I thought so. It all involves compound movements, i.e., several muscles and joints.

So when it comes to becoming more athletic, can you see that compound exercises rule? Yeah, compounds rule!

AND THE WINNER IS...

If this chapter were a boxing match, the clear winner via a unanimous decision is compound exercises. So whether it's for becoming stronger, more muscular, or developing athleticism, you can't go wrong with basing your training regimen on compound exercises. Just watch how top bodybuilder Phil Heath, basketball "king" LeBron James and elite fighters like Manny Pacquiao train for mass, strength and athleticism. They focus more on compound exercises rather than isolation ones.

THE VALUE OF ISOLATION EXERCISES

That being said, isolation exercises aren't worthless. They have high value, but only as a supplementary form of exercise rather than being the meat and potatoes of a training program or regimen.

For one, isolation exercises help provide the necessary muscular detail, which is very important for competitive body builders and fitness models. Dumbbell concentration curls help give bodybuilders the highly sought after "peak", such as those of Arnold Schwarzenegger's during his competitive days as Mr. Olympia and those of Phil Heath's, the reigning Mr. Olympia.

Another value of isolation exercises is that they can help strengthen problematic body parts. For example, some people suffer from chronic shoulder pain and some isolation shoulder exercises help strengthen the shoulder muscles and stabilize the rotator cuff, helping to manage or even relieve pain.

The rule of thumb is – especially when it comes to building muscles – is that isolation exercises are only supplementary ones that help you further refine the muscle mass you acquire via compound exercises. Never make it the bedrock of your muscle-building training program.

Chapter 5: Exercising for Muscle Growth Part III

Now that you know that compound exercises should form the bulk or foundation of your weight lifting or resistance training program, let's take a look at the best compound exercises to help you build muscle fast. These exercises offer the best bang for your muscle-building buck.

BARBELL BENCH PRESS

This is the alpha of all body building exercises in the sense that it's the one most weight lifting enthusiasts use as a barometer for measuring their strength, the basis for bragging about it, or both. While you can substitute the barbell with dumbbells, a barbell is still the best way to inflict maximum tension on your chest muscles and make them grow like crazy!

To do this, simply lie flat on a bench. Grab the barbell with a medium grip, i.e., one that allows your forearms and upper arms to make a 90-degree angle in the middle of the lift. Take the bar off the rack and with your arms locked straight, hold it above you – your beginning position.

Breathe in then start bringing the barbell down gradually until it touches your chest's middle portion. By gradually, I mean it should take about 2 seconds for the barbell to touch your middle chest from the beginning position.

After 2 seconds at the bottom, begin pushing the barbell back up to the beginning position but short of locking out your elbows. This should take you only 1 second to complete. Don't let it get to a point where your elbows lock because it will let your chest rest and reduce the optimal tension, and it will also increase your risk of injuring your elbow joints. Make sure you're breathing out as you push the barbell up – the concentric phase of the movement.

Be careful not to let the barbell go too far forward when you push it back up to minimize risk of injuries or accidents. Also, make sure that when you lower the barbell, it doesn't touch anything else other than your middle chest. And lastly, don't let the barbell bounce off your chest. Simply let it touch the middle chest and let it stay for 2 seconds before pushing back up.

This completes one repetition or rep, as weight lifting enthusiasts would like to call it. The optimal rep range for muscle building is between 8 to 12 repetitions. This means you must use a weight that allows you to complete at least 8 reps and a maximum of 12. If you can't reach 8 reps, it's too heavy. If you can make 13 reps, it's time to increase the weight. After the last rep, place the barbell back in the rack. That's 1 set. Perform 2 to 3 sets.

Feel your chest muscles contract – the lift should be done mostly by your chest and not your arms or shoulders. To ensure this, draw your shoulders back and your chest out all through out the movement. Resist the urge to push off with your shoulders so that your chest gets all the tension for optimal growth.

A word of caution though: If you're new to weight lifting, it's best to have another person spot you on your lift to minimize risk of injuries. If you can't find someone to spot you, better be safe than macho – use a lighter weight than prescribed. This is only until you get the hang of the exercise. For this purpose, you can use a weight that you can complete up to 15 reps per set.

BARBELL DEADLIFTS

This exercise primarily targets your lower back muscles. It also involves your hamstrings as support. Actually, you can do deadlifts holding 2 dumbbells – one on each side. But as with the bench there's just something about the barbell that really makes weight lifting exercises more badass and in the process, more effective for building mass.

To perform this exercise, go near the barbell that's on the floor. Place yourself in the middle of the bar with your feet hip-width apart and feet planted firmly on the ground. Then, bend at your hip to hold the barbell with your hands about shoulder-width apart. Use alternating grips to hold the barbell, i.e., one palm facing outward or forward and the other palm facing inward or backward. Power lifters typically use alternating grips for deadlifts.

As you bend, make sure that your lower back remains straight to avoid injuring it. Never perform deadlifts – or any motion that involves picking something up from the ground – with your lower back arched or hunched forward. From start to finish, always keep your lower back straight as a ruler – bending at the waist and at the knees. Bending at the waist only will make you lose balance and harder to lift the barbell to execute the movement.

With feet planted firmly on the ground, legs and waist bent, lower back straight and gripping the bar with alternate palms, it's time to lift the barbell. Pull the barbell upward using your legs and lower back, keeping the lower back straight at all times. At the top of the movement, squeeze your shoulder blades together and drive your hips to touch the barbell as it hangs from your arms. Gradually reverse the whole movement to bring the bar back to the floor, still keeping your lower back straight. That's one repetition or rep. Perform 8 to 12 reps per set and do 2 to 3 sets.

Word of caution: keep your lower back straight all the time to avoid lower back injury (same goes true for picking up a pen from the floor, etc.) and don't drop the barbell on the floor to let it bounce up for the next rep. Gradually bring down the bar until it touches the floor before lifting it up again.

BARBELL SQUATS

The bench press may be the most "prestigious" of the compound exercises but when it comes to recruiting the most number of muscles and the largest muscle groups, nothing beats the barbell squat. It also burns the most calories. If you've seen the massively cut legs of the greatest bodybuilders such as Ronnie Coleman, Jay Cutler, Dorian Yates, Phil Heath and Kai Greene, you bet that those dudes didn't build those sets of wheels (bodybuilding slang for things or legs) with machine leg presses and leg extensions. They were built using squats!

Start by placing the barbell on a rack. The height of the rack should be such that if you place your trapezius (traps) below the barbell and with your lower back straight (If you find it hard to keep your lower back straight, consider using a weightlifting belt), your knees should be bent at an angle that your body's too low on the ground but not high to the point you're practically standing up straight as the barbell rests on your traps. This is to ensure you have just the right allowance to lift the barbell up to perform the squat.

As you support the barbell with your traps, your head should face forward and your chest must be facing up. Your feet should be hip-width apart and facing outward as you need it to be. Lift the barbell off the rack, stand straight, and take a step backward to create enough space. This is the beginning position.

Start the movement by gradually bending at the knees to descend. As you do this, avoid putting your hips very far back to minimize risk of losing balance and injury. The best way to do this is by keeping your back straight and making sure that as you descend, your knees never move forward beyond your toes. This ensures you keep your torso as upright as realistically possible, which is the safest way to do squats.

How low should you go? As low as possible but without straining your knees excessively when you push back up to return to the beginning position. If your knees feel too strained and become painful, you've descended too low.

From the lowered position, use your legs to push your torso – and the barbell – back up to return to the beginning position. To maximize tension and minimize risk of injury, don't lock your knees at the top of the movement. Not only does it allow your legs to "rest" by taking off tension from the muscles to the knee joints, locking the knees puts excessive strain on them. So remember, stop short of locking out the knees to complete one rep. Perform 2 to 3 sets of 8 to 12 reps each.

BARBELL ROWS

This exercise primarily works out your middle back muscles, but it also works out your lower back, forearms, and legs as support. With the barbell on the floor, hold it using a pronated grip – both hands or palms facing down or back towards you – with knees bent and your torso forward. Again, keep your lower back straight and if you find it hard to do so at first, use a weightlifting belt at the start to help you learn how to keep your lower back straight during lifts like these. At the starting position, your lower back must already be straight and nearly parallel to the floor then lift your torso slightly upward – still keeping your lower back straight – so that the barbell is hanging from your arms.

Keeping your torso still, feet planted firmly on the ground, and lower back straight, lift the barbell up until it touches your stomach, ribs or solar plexus, depending on your angle, breathing out as you perform the movement. As you do this, keep the elbows near your body and avoid using the upper arms to lift the weight – it should be your back that must do the work. You should only use your forearms for holding the bar – letting it hang from your arms so to speak.

At the top position, hold and squeeze your back muscles for 2 seconds before lowering the barbell back to a dead hang in a controlled manner, never letting it bounce at the bottom.

Breathe in as you lower the barbell. At the bottom, it shouldn't touch the floor. This is 1 rep. Do 8 to 12 reps for 2 to 3 sets.

A word of caution though: if you have lower back problems to begin with, don't perform this exercise. Instead, use a machine such as a low pulley row to work out your lower back. While this may not be as effective as the barbell row, it will still help you build muscle mass but without the risk of aggravating your pre-existing lower back problem. Less muscle growth, but also less risk.

MILITARY OR OVERHEAD PRESSES

This particular exercise primarily targets your front shoulder muscles or front delts and works out your triceps too.

Sitting on a military press bench, the barbell should be behind your head. Adjust the height so that it isn't too low that it practically tears your rotator cuff just to lift to assume the beginning position. Grab the barbell with a pronated or forward-facing palm or grip that's slightly more than shoulder-width apart.

Lift the barbell up over your head but stop short of locking out at the elbows to minimize risk of elbow injury and maintain continuous tension on your shoulders and triceps. Then, bring the barbell down to nearly touching your collar bone (breathing in as you do) before pushing it all the way back up (exhaling as you push), stopping short of locking your arms or elbows. This is one rep. Perform 2 to 3 sets of 8 to 12 reps each.

To end the set, gradually bring the barbell down behind your head on the rack. It's best if you can have someone assist you in putting the barbell back on the rack.

Word of caution: If you have pre-existing problems with your rotator cuff, assume an alternate beginning position where the barbell is placed in front of you instead. Same steps for executing the movement.

PULL UPS AND CHIN UPS

These exercises primarily work out your middle and upper back muscles. For the pull ups, hang on sturdy bar, placing your hands wider than your shoulders and using a pronated (palms facing forward) grip. Pull your self up until your chin touches the bar. Hold the position for 1 second before lowering yourself down. That's 1 rep. Perform 8 to 12 reps of 2 to 3 sets.

To perform chin-ups, simply change your grip to a supinated one (palms facing inward) and grip about shoulder-width apart. Same movement, reps and sets as the pull up.

If you find you're not yet strong enough to perform the recommended reps and sets, you can start by using a lat pull-down machine in the gym. Same principles and movements apply.

Chapter 6: Weight Lifting Tips for Maximum Muscles

Before we end our discussion on exercising to build muscles, I will discuss some of the most important principles or guidelines when it comes weight lifting or resistance training for building muscle mass.

WARMING UP

As I mentioned earlier, building serious muscle mass requires lifting heavy weights. And if you want to maximize your heavy lifting benefits, it's best to warm up your muscles first. Keep this in mind: The heavier the weight you want to lift, the higher the number of warm-up sets you may need. Warming up doesn't just help you lift more weight, it also helps reduce your risk for tendon and ligament injuries. Those two body parts are crucial for your efforts the lift progressively heavier weights and decreased muscle mass.

So how do you warm up? Before even beginning your light weight warm up sets, it's best to brisk walk on the treadmill or around the block, or ride the stationary bicycle for 10 minutes. This helps to get your blood flowing efficiently even before you start your lightweight sets.

Then, perform one or two warm up sets you're programmed exercise using 50% to 75% of the weight you plan to use for your 2 to 3 main workout sets. The warm-up sets make your muscles limber enough and joints loose enough to handle the serious poundage you will be hoisting in your main workout sessions or sets.

WEIGHT

The most common question most weight lifting beginners ask is how much weight to lift or use? I'm pretty sure that's one of your questions as well. As much as I'd like to give you text number, only you can answer that depending on your goals.

Weightlifting goals can be strength building or muscle building. If your primary goal is to build strength, you should use a weight wherein you can only perform a maximum of 6 repetitions per set. If you're able to do more than that, it means you're using a relatively lightweight for your goal.

If your primary goal is to build up muscular endurance, you should use a weight that allows you to perform a minimum of 15 repetitions per set. Anything less than that means you're using too much weight for your goal.

But if your primary goal is to build serious muscle mass, which I assume is your goal since you're reading this book, then you should use a weight that allows you to perform a minimum of 8 reps and a maximum of 12 per set. If you find you can't complete 8 repetitions, it means you're using too much weight. But if you find you're able to perform more than 12 reps, it means you're already using a relatively lightweight per your goals.

VOLUME

Other common questions beginners ask are how long or how often to work out. Some elite bodybuilders like Ronnie Coleman spend more hours a day working out a single body part then most people do in their daily commute to and from work. Are there any bodybuilders like Dorian Yates use only one main working set where he uses an insane amount of weight and asks the help of a training partner to eke out the last remaining reps necessary to optimize muscle growth. So which is which?

For most beginners, the volume that works best is between 2 to 3 sets of a given exercise. For those who are more advanced, the recommended is between 3 to 4 sets per exercise.

The issue here really, is volume, which is a total number of repetitions and sets performed for a particular muscle group. For building muscle mass, a fairly high volume is required.

As a beginner, it's best to start with 12 sets per muscle group such as legs, back, and chest. This would be composed of 3 sets of 4 exercises on one end and 2 sets of 6 exercises on the other end. For smaller muscle groups like arms and shoulders, you may need 2 to 3 sets of 6 to 8 exercises.

These however, are guidelines, not hard and fast rules. Try them out and adjust accordingly depending on your body's response.

PROGRESSIVE OVERLOAD

You need to be aggressive when it comes to stimulating muscle growth. This is because your muscle fibers tend to adapt relatively fast to the tension or stimulus that you give them, which run the risk of quickly diminishing a particular exercise and weight's muscle growth stimulating effects. What this means is that you will need to progressively overload your muscles with heavier weights or increasing tension. Basically, one of your muscle building efforts' greatest enemies is sticking to the same amount of weight or tension for excessively long periods of time.

You can continuously overload your muscles by changing the exercises you perform, increasing the weight or tension applied to the muscles, and combining some or all of the above. The point of progressive overload is to keep your muscles from adapting well to the tension or weight you give them so that they will continue growing.

One of the ways you know when to increase the weight is if you're able to perform more reps than the maximum recommended, i.e., 12 for muscle building. Once you're able to consistently perform more than 12 reps, it's time to overload the muscle by increasing the weight. Don't overload immediately as this heightens the risk of injury. Overload only when it's time to do so. And don't increase the weight or tension dramatically! Do so in small increments until you find the ideal weight or tension that allows you to perform the ideal repetitions and sets.

SEQUENCE

In most cases, the best way to build serious muscle is to prioritize compound exercises – perform them first and isolation exercises last. It's because you can hoist the most weight at the start of your workout, when your energy level is still high. And remember, compound exercises use several muscle groups, which means you'll use a greater amount of energy compared to when you're performing isolation exercises.

Using chest as an example, perform bench presses first before the isolation exercises like dumbbell flies or the pec deck because if you perform the isolations first, you won't be able to use heavier weights for the presses later on, having pre-fatigued your chest already. Now pre-exhaustion or pre-fatigued muscles can prove to be useful in specific situations, which I'll elaborate on more later, but generally speaking, compound exercises need to go first for best results.

ISOLATION FIRST, COMPOUND SECOND

There are times that the best way to progressively overload your muscles is by starting with isolation exercises instead of compound ones. When is that? When one of the supporting muscles isn't strong enough to handle the necessary weight or tension.

Here's an example. When you find that your triceps fail before your chest does on your bench presses, you're not able to fully tax your chest for optimal growth. The solution is to pre-exhaust the chest muscles first using an isolation exercise like dumbbell flies. Doing so will fatigue your chest muscles so that you do the bench press later on, you can use a lighter weight that allows you to fatigue your chest muscles and not your triceps.

However, this is an exception and should only be used until such time the smaller, supporting muscle becomes strong enough to prioritize compound exercises over isolation ones. To ensure you don't become dependent on this, it's best for you to separately train your triceps to build strength and muscle mass to catch up with your chest on the bench press later on.

REST AND RECUPERATION

Related to volume and frequency of workouts, is the question of rest and recuperation. While it's true that working out consistently at a relatively high volume is necessary for building muscle, it is possible to over do it. Some people workout their chest muscles everyday and are very disappointed at the fact that they have nothing to show for it.

In the previous example, overtraining is evident. Remember that I wrote in chapter 2 about how muscles grow, particularly the recuperation phase? If you don't give your muscles the opportunity to rest and recuperate, they will not grow.

So how much rest is needed? The consensus among most bodybuilding experts is that you need to give a particular muscle or muscle group at least 48 hours of rest and recuperation before exercising them again if the goal is to build more muscles. This is why working out a particular muscle group everyday will not lead too muscular growth.

But what about those really big and muscular dudes who are at the gym working out everyday? Why are they as big as houses despite? Well, they may be in the gym almost every day, but each day they are working out a different body part or muscle group. On Monday, they may work out chest then on Tuesday, they work out the back muscles. On Wednesday, they may workout their leg muscles before resting on Thursday. Then on Friday, they may work out their shoulder muscles and workout arms on Saturday to complete the whole body cycle for the week. Even if they work out at the gym everyday, they still give each muscle group the opportunity to get at least 48 Hours of rest and recuperation before being worked out again.

THE SPLIT

Split training refers to scheduling your workouts in such a way that you prioritize only one body part per workout session. This is the opposite of full body workouts where you exercise all the body parts in one session.

There is much benefit to the split training routine, particularly when it comes to building muscle. For one, dedicating your workout sessions to one body part allows you to lift heavier and exercise with higher volume. That allows you to maximize the stimulation of your muscles and optimize growth.

Second, split training allows you to burn more calories on a weekly basis. Why? Because you can afford to work out everyday, with each day featuring a different body part. When all you do is full body workouts, you'll need to wait 48 hours for your muscles to recuperate before working out in the gym again. With a split routine, you can be in the gym from Monday to Friday, working out a different body part each time. That allows your muscles to still rest and recuperate for at least 48 hours.

TAKE YOUR TIME

If you'd like to maximize your workouts in order to build muscle mass, you also need to take enough rest and recovery time after every set. If you remember, you need to be able to lift as much weight as you can to stimulate muscle growth. By resting little and beginning The Next sets almost immediately or prematurely, you don't give your muscles enough time to regain strength for lifting the necessary poundage. But if you take your time in between sets, you give your muscles that chance to recover its strength to lift heavy weights in the succeeding sets.

STRIKE AN ATHLETIC POSE

Particularly when performing standing exercises, about the same posture as athletes from all sports do: An athletic stance. What this means is that your feet should be firmly planted on the ground at about shoulder width with your toes slightly pointed outward, your chest out, lower back straight with a slight backward arch, shoulders back, knees slightly bent, and your head looking ahead to the front.

Why is this position crucial for standing exercises? It's because this posture is a naturally stable and strong one that is an ideal starting position for most, if not all, standing exercises.

USE A BELT

Most people you see in the gym don't use weight or lifting belts. Why? Frankly, they don't look cool. But is it also a coincidence that those people don't look as muscular as you want to be? I don't think so.

You see, you'll need to lift heavy poundage if you want to build muscle mass. But to minimize your risks for injury when lifting really heavy weights especially with exercises that involve the lower back like the deadlift and squats, you'll need the support of a good lifting belt. It's not a coincidence that the world's strongest – and most muscular, if I may add – people use weight lifting belts to support the heavy weight they hoist around.

STABILITY AND BALANCE

Have you ever seen someone perform bicep curls in the gym as if he or she is standing on a surfboard? Now that's dangerous. While we emphasize lifting heavy weights to build muscle, it shouldn't come at the expense safety. And one way to ensure safety is to perform exercises on stable ground and with a stable posture. Leave the surfing on the beach.

GRIP

Remember the point of progressive overload, which is to "confuse" your muscle fibers and prevent them from becoming too familiar with the stimulus you apply? Well, another way you can mix things up to keep your muscles from adapting is changing your grip or the way you hold the weights.

For example, if you've been performing bench presses with slightly wider than shoulder width grip, try closing the gap and utilize a shoulder-width grip to change things up. Some bodybuilders, though I'm not in favor of it, do reverse grip bench presses, where their palms face inward instead of the usual pronated or forward facing orientation. Why? Changing grips can provide new stimulus to muscle fibers for more growth.

WRAPS AND STRAPS

And speaking of grip, if you find that your grip strength is not yet at par for the weight you need to lift to tax your target muscles completely, you can use wraps or straps. There's no shame in using them. You can gradually work on your grip strength on forearm training days so you don't have to compromise the quality of your workouts that involve gripping the weights. Again, most bodybuilders use straps to build the muscle mass they have. Why shouldn't you? After all, you're goal is to build muscle, right? For as long as you don't violate anyone's rights, go for straps when needed!

DUMBBENEFITS

While I – and countless many others – have extolled the virtues of the barbell, it doesn't mean you should ignore using dumbbells. Dumbbells give your workout repertoire more variety and can help stimulate muscle fibers even more to maximize your muscle growth.

One of the benefits is angle. With barbells, you are constricted to a particular angle range but with dumbbells, you can pretty much rotate the thing however you want. Take the bench press for example. If you use a barbell, your arms must be aligned horizontally and vertically, otherwise the barbell will be unbalanced and increase the risk of injury. With dumbbells, it's ok if your left hand is angled slightly different.

Another benefit of dumbbells is that they allow your relatively problematic body parts to take a less painful position. Take for example the wrist. If you use a barbell for bench press and you have a problematic left wrist that is painful at the angle forced by the barbell, you can't twist your wrist to a comfortable one. With dumbbells, you can.

And last but not the least, the ability to control the tilt and angle allows dumbbells to stimulate your muscle fibers in many different ways. That makes it the perfect complement to barbells.

Still, the foundation of your heavy lifts need to be barbells to optimize muscle growth. Use dumbbells as your primary source of exercise if barbells prove to be problematic for you.

USE YOUR ILLUSION

No, I am not talking about that classic, best-selling double album by the immortal rock band Guns N' Roses. I'm talking about creating the illusion of creating the look of the most sought after look in bodybuilding and fitness in general – the

V-Taper. That's a look where you have wide shoulders and narrow waist.

The V-Taper is largely dependent on genetics. Having naturally broad shoulders (wide shoulder blades) and tiny waist (and hip bones), make it very easy to have that look. But how about if you have narrow shoulder bones and wide hip bones?

You can use weights to increase your shoulder muscle mass – especially the side delts – to make your shoulders wide enough to make your wide hips look relatively small. After all, the V-Taper look is all about proportions – the proportion of your shoulders to your waist and hips! That's how you can use your illusion to achieve that V-Taper look!

CHEATING IS GOOD

Now before you judge me, I'm not talking about cheating on your spouse, on your tests or in your taxes! I'm talking about cheat reps or repetitions! This s just about the only cheating in the world that I agree to!

What is a cheat rep? It's a repetition that you can't possibly complete on your own – you'll need assistance either from your spotter or via momentum to complete that rep. But cheat reps should only be used after you've already completed your required number of reps. Cheat reps should merely augment honest or properly executed reps and not take their primary place.

For example, you're already done with the 12th rep of your last set on the bench press and you can't complete another one using proper form or on your own. You can cheat 1 or 2 more reps by letting your spotter assist you just enough for you to push the barbell one or two more times. You can also use momentum to quickly push the barbell up.

THE NEED FOR SPEED

Speaking of cheat reps, I mentioned using momentum to aid you get the extra push. You gain momentum by using an explosive movement or by speeding up the movement. Speed builds momentum and in situations where cheat reps are needed, speed doesn't kill – it builds!

Just keep in mind that speed doesn't mean uncontrolled bursts of movement. Controlled speed is what can help you eke out those extra reps that can help maximize your muscle building.

DROP IT

When I say drop it, I don't mean that you try to act all macho in the gym by screaming after a really hard set and dropping the barbell or dumbbells to attract attention. When I say drop it, I am referring to the use of drop sets, which can give you a muscle burn like you've never felt before.

Drop sets are continuous sets with no rest. Drop sets are usually done as the final set of a specific exercise. In a drop set, you complete the last regular set then perform 1 to 3 more sets at progressively lighter weight. If you used 100 pounds on the last set of your bench press for example, you immediately do another set of 12 reps using 80 pounds, and another set right after using 60 pounds for the final set of the drop set. If you want to take it further, do 2 more sets at 40 and 20 pounds!

Drop sets aren't meant to be done all the time. For one, it can give you one nasty muscle burn that most mortals can't stand. Also, it's meant to be a way to bust out of plateaus and as such, it's ability to stimulate stagnating muscles lie in its limited use. If used frequently, your muscle fibers may get used to it and thus, rob you of a very effective "shock treatment" for muscle growth.

SUPERSETS

Supersets refer to working out opposing or antagonistic muscles one right after the other. For example, right after you complete a set of bench press (chest), you immediately perform a set of barbell rows (back), which constitutes one super set. The benefit of this is that you can jack up the strength on the second exercised body part, the back in our example. Just keep in mind that like the drop sets, this is ideally meant to be more of a supplementary regimen, rather than the main course.

Why? Because it's a very taxing workout and doing it very often may lead to overtraining.

Other good superset combinations include biceps and triceps, and thighs and hamstrings.

DON'T START FROM THE START

If you look at deadlifts, it's different from all the other exercises in that you begin the movement from a dead stop – without the benefit of momentum or elastic energy. Take the bench press for example. You start the movement after you lower the bar to your chest and as you lowered it, you enjoyed the benefit of the assistance of elastic energy because you didn't start from a dead stop. With the deadlift, it's much harder because the movement starts by your picking the barbell up from the floor – a dead stop! No momentum or elastic energy to start with. It's purely your muscles – it's purely you!

So what's my point? It's this: one way to change things up is to start your other exercises from a complete dead stop. Take for example again, the bench press. Instead of starting the movement by bringing down the barbell or dumbbells down to your chest, start the movement from the bottom! If you're using a barbell, lower the safety rack so that it's about 12 inches above your chest, which robs you of the chance to use elastic energy or momentum. That way, you practically start from a dead stop. You started not at the start but at nearly the bottom end. Doing this is another great way to "shock" your muscles, which makes it a great supplementary method of lifting weights for muscle building.

CHAINS AND BANDS

For many people, using chains and powerlifting bands aren't worth it. But realize that using such contraptions can give your muscle-building efforts a significant boost, especially if you use them sporadically. They help "shock" your muscles every now and then to help you bust out of muscle building plateaus.

Chains and bands are unique in that they give you variable or dynamic resistance throughout the execution of a movement. How?

Take for example weighted dips for triceps and lower chest. As you begin the movement from below, you're just using your body weight. But as you push up, you pull the chain or band that's attached to the weight and consequently pull the weight up – increasing the weight or tension during the latter part of your triceps dip movement. Now that's a unique way to stimulate muscle growth!

PYRAMIDING

No, this is not a scam. I'm talking about an approach to working out. It's an approach to working sets where the succeeding sets use heavier weights but fewer reps, hence the pyramid reference. So instead of doing 3 sets of the same reps and same weight (say 100 pounds), you can mix things up by doing 12 reps at 100 pounds for the first, 8 reps at 110 pounds for the second, and 6 reps at 120 pounds for the last and final working set.

This has the benefit of helping you become stronger, which will let you lift heavier weights at the recommended rep range for building muscle. But use this as a supplement, when you notice that you're not progressing like you used to in terms of building muscle.

PUMP IT UP

Some bodybuilders recommend using high volume (high rep, many sets) for maximum recruitment of muscle fibers, believing that anything less means you're not exerting enough effort to build muscle. Is this true or not?

The answer is – it depends. When you look at two of the greatest bodybuilders ever to walk the planet – Dorian Yates and Ronnie Coleman – they have contrasting styles. Dorian Yates' approach was low volume, heavy weights. Ronnie Coleman on the other hand, used a high volume approach, still with heavy weights. Some people respond better to the Dorian Yates approach. Others respond to the Ronnie Coleman approach. You'll need to figure out what's best for you.

However, you should only consider this once you've already gotten enough weight lifting or training experience. As a beginner, focus on getting the basics first. After several months of consistent muscular gains, try to increase volume to amp up the results.

TWO IS BETTER THAN ONE

Having a training partner who is also after the same goal of building muscles can be a great plus to your own efforts. Why? You can encourage and challenge each other when working out. When working out alone, there's a tendency to lose interest because of boredom or get discouraged if you're stuck at a certain point. But when you have a partner, you can be encouraged and even challenged to try different things and lift heavier weights to help you bust out of your plateau. Plus, a training partner can help you eke out those much needed cheat reps.

Just make sure your partner is a responsible one who focused on the goal at hand: building muscle. Otherwise, that person may just be a source of distraction, in which case it may be better to work out alone. But generally speaking, a training partner's an asset in your muscle building efforts.

Chapter 7: Eating for Muscle Growth

Now that we covered training and rest/recuperation, we will end by discussing the most taken forgotten member of the muscle-building trinity: nutrition.

MACRONUTRIENTS

A calorie isn't just a calorie – it's either carbohydrates, fat or protein. Carbohydrates act as the body's main fuel source for working out. In particular, it becomes glycogen – your muscles readily available source of energy. Protein acts as the main building block of muscle cells – think of it as the raw materials by which muscle fibers repair themselves and increase in number. Without adequate protein, you won't just fail to gain muscle mass but you may lose it as well. Fats are primarily for special bodily functions like utilization of certain nutrients as well as for protection of internal organs. It's also a good source of energy but not as readily available or as clean as carbohydrates.

PROTEIN FOR MUSCLE GROWTH

So how much is enough for muscle growth? Most experts agree on an average of 1 to 1.5 grams of protein per pound of bodyweight daily. This means if you weigh 150 pounds, you'll need to consume between 150 to 225 grams of protein daily in conjunction with a good weight lifting or resistance training program if you want to build serious muscle mass.

More than just the daily portions, you also need to consider the frequency of eating those grams of protein. When I say 150 grams a day, I don't mean you can eat them all in just one sitting. You'll need to eat it across 5 to 6 smaller meals a day. Why?

First, your body can only consume, process and synthesize a certain amount of calories – be it carbohydrates, protein or fat – in one sitting. The excess will simply be stored as body fat. When you divide your calories across 5 to 6 smaller meals a day, spaced about 2 to 3 hours apart, you give your body the opportunity to make full use of those calories. If you don't believe me, why do you think bodybuilders, fitness competitors and fitness models eat many small meals a day?

So what does each meal look like? It should be a good combination of complex carbohydrates, lean protein, and some fat. The easiest way to check your portions is this: fist-sized serving for carbohydrates, palm sized serving for protein, and thumb sized serving for fat.

If you want to be very anal about it, you can check out calorie counters to find very good sources of lean protein and know how much to eat daily. For starters, the best sources of lean protein include skinless chicken and turkey breasts, tuna, and egg whites.

OF PROTEIN SUPPLEMENTS

If you find it hard to gulp down that much meat for protein, don't worry. Bodybuilders, fitness models and competitors also feel the same way and as such, they supplement their protein needs with protein shakes. These are easy and delicious ways of getting in your protein requirements daily.

Protein shakes come in two general forms: whey and casein. Their difference is like the difference between simple and complex carbohydrates. Whey protein is fast acting, i.e., easily digested, broken down and absorbed by the muscles. Casein on the other hand is like complex carbohydrates – they're slower to digest, break down and be synthesized into the muscles.

So which is better? Well, it depends. Whey protein is great as a pre or post workout source of protein because you need immediate proteins before, during and right after your lifting sessions. Casein on the other hand, is perfect for days and times you're not working out. In fact, it's perfect as a nighttime shake because it provides your muscles with a steady stream of quality protein during the night when you're asleep.

POST WORKOUT CARBS

Right after you finish working out, it's crucial to replenish your glycogen stores, which you've depleted significantly during workouts. You have a 2-hour window to do this by consuming simple or quick acting carbs. So if you have a sweet tooth, the best time to indulge is right after a workout session. Because the body needs to replenish glycogen stores, the chances are much higher that simple carbs like sugar will be converted into glycogen for storage in your muscles instead of body fat. Your ability to recover and recuperate your worked out muscles will be highly dependent on your ability to provide it with both fast acting protein and carbs.

Conclusion

Congratulations! You are now armed with enough knowledge to start building your muscles and hit the beach looking really good and strong come the summertime. Or if you're an athlete who needs more muscles for better performance, be ready to bring your physical condition and game to a higher level.

However, all the things you learned here will just be trivia if you don't apply them. As such, I highly encourage you to start acting on what you learned immediately! You don't have to apply everything – take baby steps. Enroll in a gym first. Next, hire an instructor. Finally, show up for your first workout sessions. The important thing is you start moving by applying what you learned, one baby step at a time.

I also advise applying everything all in one sitting. You'll run the risk of overtraining, which can either make you quit or worse, get injured. Again, take one step at a time. The important thing is you continue building momentum so that you become practically unstoppable in your muscle-building efforts.

Thank you and good luck!

www.ingramcontent.com/pod-product-compliance
Lightning Source LLC
Chambersburg PA
CBHW070035040426
42333CB00040B/1687